Anti-Inflammatory Diet

The Comprehensive Beginners Guide To Dealing With
Inflammation And Changing Your Life

(The Step By Step Guide To Detoxify And Cleanse The Body And Increase Energy)

Andres Erickson

TABLE OF CONTENTS

Introduction..1

Organic Asparagus Recipe...3

Zucchini Salad 4

Avocado Wrapped In Bacon 6

Vegetable Skewers And Grilled Cheese 8

Tasty Turkey Baked Balls 10

Baked Pork Chops With Cashew...........................12

Cranberry Pork..14

Chicken, Corn & Spinach Sauté.............................16

Sprouts & Slices In Wheat Wrap..........................18

Feta-Filled & Tomato-Topped Turkey Burger Bites..20

Simply Sautéed Flaky Fillet....................................22

Spicy Sautéed Chinese Chicken 24

Pork With Mushrooms And Cucumbers............26

Oregano Pork 29

Wild Rice With Spicy Chickpeas.............................31

Seafood Salad And Salsa Verde With Thai Basil 34

Cashew Pesto & Parsley With Veggies 37

Creamy Pork And Tomatoes....................................40

Pork With Balsamic Fresh Onion Sauce 42

Ground Pork Pan 45

Tasty Thai Chicken In Crisp Cups..........................48

Zesty Zucchini & Chicken In Classic Santa Fe Stir-Fry...50

Crispy Cheese-Crusted Fish Fillet 52

Ambrosial Avocado & Salmon Salad In Lemon-Dressed Layers 54

Sautéed Shrimp Jambalaya Jumble......................57

Toasted Tilapia Topped With Panko & Pecans 59

Tortilla Tostadas With Peppered Potato & Kingly Kale..61

- Vanilla Turmeric Orange Juice 64
- Hibiscus Ginger Gelatin 66
- Buckwheat And Sweet Potatoes 68
- Zucchini Patties 70
- Shrimp Mix 72
- Spinach And Lentils Stew 73
- Sweet Potato Mix 75
- Pea Stew 78
- Green Beans Stew 80
- Chickpeas Salad 81
- Quinoa And Beans 83
- Cucumber And Green Fresh Onion S Salad 85
- Barley And Kale 86
- Herbed Mango Mix 88
- Cabbage Slaw 90
- Cucumber With Apples Alad 92
- Parsley Avocado Mix 93
- Endives And Broccoli 95

Arugula Salad 97

Morning Bowl.. 100

30 2. Breakfast Stir Fry 102

Cereal Nibs 105

Chicken Muffins... 107

Egg Porridge 109

Celery Root Hash Browns 111

Zucchini Pasta With Avocado Sauce................. 112

Blueberry Chia Pudding... 114

Collard Green Wrap... 115

Zucchini Garlic Fries.. 118

Mashed Cauliflower... 119

Conclusion 121

Introduction

What is Inflammation?

In the simplest terms, Inflammation is the process of how the body's immune system reacts whenever it detects the presence of a foreign entity inside the body or any form of injury. During an inflammatory response, White Blood Cells alongside a number of different substances tries to protect the body from further damage that might result from the contamination.

However, things change when this very action takes a turn for the worst.

Whenever you are dealing with something such as Arthritis, which is also related to chronic inflammation, the defense mechanism of the body seems to malfunction and trigger an inflammatory response even though there are no contamination.

Diseases that tend to do these are largely known as "Auto Immune" diseases and instead of protecting the body, the body's own auto-immune system starts to harm itself and damage the tissues

That being said, let's have a look at some of the main reasons of Inflammation.

Organic Asparagus Recipe

Ingredients:

Unrefined sea salt

Pepper to taste

2 pound of asparagus

2 tbsp. buttered with grass (melted)

Directions:

1. Cut asparagus, this is easily accomplished by breaking off the ends where it naturally breaks off.
2. Pour the melted butter over asparagus and toss for coating.
3. Season generously with salt and pepper.

4. Place on a hot grill and grill for about 6 -25 minutes until the asparagus is soft.

Zucchini Salad

Ingredients:

- 35 g fresh basil
- 25 g of fresh mint
- 280 g burrata
- 2 zucchini
- 4 tablespoons mild olive oil
- 2 tbsp. balsamic vinegar
- 70 g of hazelnuts

Directions:

1. Cut the zucchini into 2 cm long slices. Season with salt and pepper and sprinkle with olive oil, heat the electric smoker and smoke the zucchini slices in 4 minutes. Turn

halfway. Put the zucchini slices in a bowl, mix with the balsamic vinegar and let stand until use.
2. Heat a pan without oil or butter and roast the hazelnuts until golden brown for 8 minutes over medium heat. Cool on a plate and chop roughly.
3. Cut basil leaves and mint roughly. The stems of basil finely chop; they have a lot of taste. Mix the zucchini with the herbs and the rest of the oil. Tear the burrata to pieces.
4. Divide first the zucchini and then the burrata over the plates. Sprinkle with the roasted hazelnuts and herbs - season with (freshly ground) pepper and possibly salt.

Avocado Wrapped In Bacon

Ingredients:

2 6 -25 strips of bacon

2 avocados (ripe)

Directions:

1. For the avocado wrapped in bacon wrapped in bacon, first, Preheat your electric smoker to 250 °F.
2. Halve the avocado and remove the kernel. Carefully remove the pulp
3. Then cut lengthwise into approximately 2 cm thick slits.

4. Wrap each column with a strip of bacon and place on the baking sheet.
5. Put the avocado wrapped in bacon in the smoker until the bacon is crispy.
6. Best observe because every oven is a little different.

Vegetable Skewers And Grilled Cheese

Ingredients:

- 250 g (1 lb.) whole white mushrooms
- 45 ml (2 tablespoons) of olive oil
- 25 ml (2 teaspoons) balsamic vinegar
- (1 teaspoon) of dried oregano
- 2 colored peppers, seeded and cut into cubes
- 4 45 g (1/2 lbs) Halloumi type grilled cheese, cubed

Directions:

1. Preheat the barbecue to medium-high power. Oil the grill.
2. In a bowl, mix all the ingredients. Salt and pepper.

3. Thread the vegetables alternately on skewers.
4. Thread the cheese on other skewers. Reserve on a large plate.
5. Grill the vegetable for 25 minutes, turning them a few times during cooking with tongs.
6. Oil the grate again.
7. Grill the cheese skewers on both sides, turning them over as soon as the cheese begins to grill, about 2 minute on each side.
8. Serve immediately. Serve with pita bread, if desired.

Tasty Turkey Baked Balls

Ingredients:

3 pound ground turkey

1 cup fresh breadcrumbs, white or whole wheat

3 Tbsp parsley, freshly chopped

4 -Tbsps milk or water

A dash of salt and pepper

A pinch of freshly grated nutmeg

1 cup Parmesan cheese, freshly grated

1 Tbsp basil, freshly chopped

1 Tbsp oregano, freshly chopped

3 pc large egg, beaten

Directions:

1. Preheat your oven to 480 °F. Line two baking pans with parchment paper.
2. Stir in all of the ingredients in a large mixing bowl. Form 3 inch balls from the mixture and place each ball in the baking pan.
3. Put the pan in the oven.
4. Bake for 45 minutes, or until the turkey cooks through and the surfaces turn brown.
5. Turn the meatballs once halfway into the cooking.

Baked Pork Chops With Cashew

Ingredients:

2 teaspoons garlic powder

A pinch of salt and black pepper

5 teaspoon smoked paprika

2 teaspoon chipotle chili powder

4 pork chops

2 fresh eggs, whisked

1 cup cashew meal

1/2 cup sunflower seeds, minced

Directions:

1. In a bowl, mix the cashew meal with sunflower seeds, garlic powder, salt, pepper, paprika, and chili powder.
2. Dip the pork chops in whisked fresh eggs, then in cashew mix and place them on a lined baking sheet and bake at 450 degrees F for 35 minutes.
3. Divide between plates and serve.

Cranberry Pork

Ingredients:

7 pound pork roast

1 teaspoon fresh grated ginger

2 tablespoon coconut flour

A pinch of mustard powder

A pinch of salt and black pepper

1 cup cranberries

1/2 cup water

Juice of 1 fresh Lemon

2 garlic cloves, minced

Directions:

1. In your slow cooker, mix the roast with the ginger, flour, mustard, salt, pepper, cranberries, water, fresh Lemon juice, and garli
2. Cover then cook on low temperature for at least 8-8 ½ hours. Slice and divide everything between plates and serve.

Chicken, Corn & Spinach Sauté

Ingredients:

3 tsp cumin

4 cups baby spinach leaves

Juice of one lime

1/2 cup goat cheese, crumbled

Salt and pepper, to taste

3 Tbsp olive oil

3 clove garlic, minced

4 pc chicken breasts, sliced

1 cup corn kernels

3 pc zucchini, cubed

Directions:

1. Sauté the chicken with garlic and olive oil in a skillet placed over medium high heat Cook for about a minute until the chicken turns brown. Remove the chicken from the pan. Set aside.
2. In the same skillet, add in the corn and zucchini, and cook for a minute until the zucchini is tender. Add the cumin, and stir while cooking further for one more minute.
3. Put the browned chicken back into the skillet, and cook until done. Stir in the lime juice and spinach, and keep cooking until the spinach wilts. Sprinkle with salt and pepper.
4. Just before serving, stir in the goat cheese.

Sprouts & Slices In Wheat Wrap

Ingredients:

1/2 cup tomatoes, diced

1/7 cup red fresh onion s, diced

1/2 cup mozzarella, partly skimmed, shredded

1/2 cup hummus or guacamole dressing

3 pc whole-wheat wrap, large

1/2 cup carrots, grated

1 cup romaine lettuce, shredded

1 pc cucumber, sliced round, then halved

1 cup bean sprouts

Directions:

1. In a medium-sized mixing bowl, prepare the dressing or spread by combining all of the ingredients excluding the cheese and wrap. Mix well until thoroughly combined.
2. On a clean table, spread out the whole-wheat wrap.
3. Spread the dressing evenly on the wrap. Be sure to leave a couple of inches on one end of the wrap for folding.
4. Add the cheese to an even layer over the spread.
5. Fold over the full wrap and tuck in at the bottom.

Feta-Filled & Tomato-Topped Turkey Burger Bites

Ingredients:

1 cup tomatoes, sun-dried, diced

1 cup Feta cheese, low fat

4 Tbsps green fresh onion s or chives, diced

3 lb turkey, lean, ground

1 tsp black pepper

Kosher or sea salt to taste

Directions:

1. Stir in all the listed ingredients in a mixing bowl.

2. Mix well until blended thoroughly.
3. Divide the mixture evenly into four patties. Store them in the refrigerator.
4. When cooking time comes, you can either grill or fry the frozen patties for about 25 minutes each on both sides.
5. Serve by topping the burgers with your preferred condiments.

Simply Sautéed Flaky Fillet

Ingredients:

3 pc lemon, juice

Salt and pepper to taste

1/2 cup parsley or cilantro, chopped

10 fillets tilapia

4 Tbsps olive oil

Directions:

1. Sauté tilapia fillets with olive oil in a medium-sized skillet placed over medium heat.
2. Cook for 4 minutes on each side until the fish flakes easily with a fork.
3. Add salt and pepper to taste. Pour the fresh Lemon juice to each fillet.
4. To serve, sprinkle the cooked fillets with chopped parsley or cilantro.

Spicy Sautéed Chinese Chicken

Ingredients:

3 Tbsp ginger, peeled and minced

3 Tbsp garlic-chili sauce or chili paste

3 Tbsp Hoisin sauce

3 Tbsp light soy sauce

For the Chicken:

3 lb chicken breasts, boneless, skinless, cubed

6 Tbsps canola oil

Directions:

1. Whisk all the marinade ingredients altogether in a mixing bowl.
2. Add in the chicken pieces, and toss lightly to coat the chicken uniformly with the marinade.
3. Cover the bowl. Chill in the refrigerator for 25 minutes.
4. Sauté the chicken pieces with canola oil in a medium-sized pan placed over medium high heat.
5. Cook for about 10 minutes until its juices run clear and cook through.
6. To serve, place the cooked chicken over a choice of either cooked quinoa or brown rice noodles, or brown rice.

Pork With Mushrooms And Cucumbers

Ingredients:

Juice of 2 lime

1/2 cup cilantro, chopped

Pinch of sea salt

Pinch black pepper

2 cup white mushrooms, halved

2 tablespoons balsamic vinegar

2 tablespoons olive oil

1 teaspoon oregano, dried

4 pork chops

2 garlic cloves, minced

Directions:

1. Warm a pan with the oil on medium heat, add the pork chops and brown for 2 minutes on each side.
2. Put the rest of the ingredients, toss, cook on medium heat for 25 minutes, divide between plates and serve.

Oregano Pork

Ingredients:

2 tablespoon sweet paprika

2 teaspoon fresh onion powder

2 tablespoons chili powder

2 garlic cloves, minced

A pinch of salt and black pepper

2 pounds pork roast, sliced

2 tablespoons oregano, chopped

1/2 cup balsamic vinegar

2 cup tomato paste

Directions:

1. In your slow cooker, combine the roast with the oregano, the vinegar, and the other ingredients, toss, put the lid on and cook on Low for 8 hours.
2. Divide everything between plates and serve.

Wild Rice With Spicy Chickpeas

Ingredients:

1/2 Cup sunflower oil

4 Cups chickpeas

2 tsp Flour

2 tsp Curry powder

4 tsp Paprika powder

2 tsp Dill

4 tbsp parsley (chopped)

2 Medium fresh onion (thinly sliced)

2 Cups currants

2 Cup basmati rice

2 Cup wild rice

Salt & pepper to taste

4tbsp Olive oil

2 tbsp Garlic powder

2tsp cumin powder

Directions:

1. For cooking wild rice, fill the half pot with water and bring it to boil.
2. Put the rice and let it simmer for at least 45 minutes.
3. Take olive in the pot and heat it on medium flame.
4. Now add cumin powder, salt, and water and bring it to boil.
5. Then add basmati rice and cook for 25 minutes.
6. Leave rice for cooking and prepare spicy chickpeas.

7. Heat 2tbsp of olive oil in the pan and toss chickpeas, garlic powder, salt & pepper, cumin, and paprika powder in it.
8. In another pan, cook fresh onion with sunflower oil until it is golden brown and add flour.
9. Mix flour and fresh onion with your hands.
10. For serving, place both types of rice in a bowl with spicy chickpeas and fry the fresh onion .
11. Garnish it with parsley and herbs.

Seafood Salad And Salsa Verde With Thai Basil

Ingredients:

35 ml (2 tablespoon) lime juice

25 ml (2 teaspoons) fish sauce (nuoc-mam)

2 teaspoons (25 mL) turmeric

2 bulb of fennel, thinly sliced with mandolin

450 g (2 cups) baby potatoes, cooked

2 green fresh onion s, chopped

2 tomato, quartered

Thai basil leaves, to taste

45 g (2 cup) Thai basil leaves

45 g (2 cup) coriander leaves

1/2 cup (60 mL) vegetable oil

46 ml (4 tablespoons) lime juice

45 ml (2 tablespoons) of water

2 green fresh onion , cut into sections

Seafood and vegetables

10 00 g (2 lbs) of mussels, cleaned

250 g (1 lbs) medium shrimp (4 3 40), shelled and deveined

4 small squid, trimmed

35 ml (2 tablespoon) vegetable oil

Directions:
1. Salsa Verde
2. In the electric smoker, finely grind all the ingredients.
3. Seafood and vegetables
4. Preheat the electric smoker to 250 °F.

5. In a large bowl, combine mussels, shrimp, squid, oil, lime juice, fish sauce and turmeriSalt and pepper.
6. Place the mussels directly on the electric smoker. Close it and cook the mussels until they are all open. Discard those that remain closed. Place in a bowl. Shell the mussels (keep some for service, if desired).
7. Grill shrimp and squid for 2 to 8 minutes per side or until shrimp and squid are cooked and browned. On a work surface, cut squid into 2 cm (1 inch) slices. Book.
8. Place the fennel in a bowl. Lightly oil, then season with salt and pepper.
9. Spread seafood and vegetables on plates. Sprinkle salsa Verde and garnish with Thai basil leaves.

Cashew Pesto & Parsley With Veggies

Ingredients:

4 Zucchini (sliced)

8 Soaked bamboo skewers

2 Red capsicums

1/2 Cup olive oil

900 grams Eggplant

4 Fresh Lemon cheeks

For Serving

Couscous salad

For Preparing Cashew Pesto

1 Cup cashew (roasted)

1 Cup parsley

2 Cup grated parmesan

2tbsp Lime juice

1/2 Cup olive oil

Directions:

1. Toss capsicum, eggplant, and zucchini with oil and salt and thread it onto skewers.
2. Cook bamboo sticks for 3 hours on a barbecue grill pan on medium heat.
3. Also, grill fresh Lemon cheeks from both sides.
4. For preparing cashew pesto, combine all ingredients in the food processor and blend.
5. For serving, place grill skewers in a plate with grill fresh Lemon slices and drizzle some cashew pesto over it.

Creamy Pork And Tomatoes

Ingredients:

2 jalapeno pepper, chopped

Pinch of sea salt

Pinch of black pepper

2 tablespoon hot pepper

2 tablespoons fresh Lemon juice

2 pounds pork stew meat, cubed

2 tablespoons avocado oil

2 cup tomatoes, cubed

2 cup coconut cream

2 tablespoon mint, chopped

Directions:

1. Warm a pan with the oil over medium heat, add the meat and brown for 10 minutes.
2. Add the rest of the ingredients, toss, cook over medium heat for 45 minutes more, divide between plates and serve.

Pork With Balsamic Fresh Onion Sauce

Ingredients:

2 pounds pork roast, sliced

2 tablespoons balsamic vinegar

1 cup vegetable stock

Pinch of sea salt

Pinch black pepper

2 yellow fresh onion , chopped

4 scallions, chopped

2 tablespoons avocado oil

2 tablespoon rosemary, chopped

2 tablespoon fresh Lemon zest, grated

Directions:

1. Warm a pan with the oil on medium heat, add the fresh onion , and the scallions and sauté for 10 minutes.
2. Add the rest of the ingredients except the meat, stir, and simmer for 10 minutes.
3. Add the meat, toss gently, cook over medium heat for 35 minutes, divide between plates and serve.

Ground Pork Pan

Ingredients:

2 tomato, cubed

1 cup mushrooms, halved

Pinch of sea salt

Pinch black pepper

2 tablespoon basil, chopped

2 tablespoons coconut aminos

2 garlic cloves, minced

2 red chilies, chopped

2 tablespoons olive oil

2 pounds pork stew meat, ground

2 red bell pepper, chopped

2 green bell pepper, chopped

Directions:

1. Warm a pan with the oil on medium heat, add the garlic, chilies, bell peppers, tomato, and the mushrooms and sauté for 10 minutes.
2. Add the meat and the rest of the ingredients, toss, cook over medium heat for 25 minutes more, divide between plates and serve.

Tasty Thai Chicken In Crisp Cups

Ingredients:

3 Tbsp fish sauce

1 pc lime, juiced

3 tsp soy sauce, reduced-sodium

3 head iceberg lettuce, separated into cups

A handful of cilantro and mint, finely chopped

6 Tbsps cooking oil

1 lb chicken breast, ground

4 pcs shallots, diced

1/2 pc red fresh onion , diced

3 clove garlic, finely minced

Jalapeño or Fresno chilies, freshly minced

Directions:

1. Sauté the ground chicken with a tablespoon of olive oil in a large wok placed over high heat. Cook for about 8 minutes until the surfaces of the ground chicken turn brown.
2. Push the browned ground chicken to one side of the wok, and pour in the remaining oil. Add in the shallots, red fresh onion , garlic, and fresh chilies.
3. Sauté these added ingredients for about half a minute until effusing their fragrance. Pour in the sauce, juice of one lime, and soy sauce.
4. Stir the entire mixture, including the ground chicken until cooked thoroughly.
5. To serve, distribute the cooked mixture evenly in lettuce cups.

Zesty Zucchini & Chicken In Classic Santa Fe Stir-Fry

Ingredients:

3 tsp paprika, smoked

3 tsp cumin, ground

1 tsp chili powder

1/2 tsp sea salt

4 Tbsp fresh lime juice

1/2 cup cilantro, freshly chopped

3 Tbsp olive oil

4 pcs chicken breasts, sliced

3 pc fresh onion , small, diced

4 cloves garlic, minced

3 pc zucchini, diced

1 cup carrots, shredded

Brown rice or quinoa, when serving

Directions:

1. Sauté the chicken with olive oil for about 8 minutes until the chicken turns brown. Set aside.
2. Use the same wok and add the fresh onion and garliCook until the fresh onion is tender.
3. Add in the carrots and zucchini. Stir the mixture, and cook further for about a minute. Add all the seasonings into the mix, and stir to cook for another minute.
4. Return the chicken in the wok, and pour in the lime juice. Stir to cook until everything cooks through.

5. To serve, place the mixture over cooked rice or quinoa and top with the freshly chopped cilantro.

Crispy Cheese-Crusted Fish Fillet

Ingredients:

1/2 tsp sea salt

1/2 tsp ground pepper

3 Tbsp olive oil

4-pcs tilapia fillets

1/2 cup whole-wheat breadcrumbs

1/2 cup Parmesan cheese, grated

Directions:

1. Preheat the oven to 480°F.

2. Stir in the breadcrumbs, Parmesan cheese, salt, pepper, and olive oil in a mixing bowl. Mix well until blended thoroughly.
3. Coat the fillets with the mixture, and lay each on a lightly sprayed baking sheet.
4. Place the sheet in the oven. Bake for 25 minutes until the fillets cook through and turn brownish.

Ambrosial Avocado & Salmon Salad In Lemon-Dressed Layers

Ingredients:

For the Avocado & Salmon Salad:

2 Tbsp olive oil, extra-virgin

2 tsp honey

1/7 tsp Kosher or sea salt

1/7 tsp black pepper

1 tsp Dijon mustard

4-units jars

10 oz wild salmon

3 pc avocado, pitted, peeled, and diced

4 cups loosely packed salad greens

1 cup Monterey Jack cheese, reduced-fat, shredded

¾-cup tomato, chopped

3 Tbsp fresh Lemon juice, freshly squeezed

For the Fresh Lemon Dressing:

2 Tbsp fresh Lemon juice, freshly squeezed

Directions:

1. Combine and whisk all the dressing ingredients excluding the olive oil in a small mixing bowl. Mix well.
2. Drizzle gradually with the oil into the dressing mixture, and keep whisking while pouring.

3. Pour the dressing as to distribute evenly into each jar.
4. Distribute uniformly into each jar similar amounts of the following ingredients in this order: diced tomatoes, cheese, avocado, salmon, and lettuce.
5. Secure each jar by with its lid, and chill the jars in the fridge until ready for serving.

Sautéed Shrimp Jambalaya Jumble

Ingredients:

25 oz. medium shrimp, peeled

1/2 cup celery, chopped

1 cup fresh onion , chopped

3 Tbsp oil or butter

1/2 tsp garlic, minced

1/2 tsp fresh onion salt or sea salt

1/4 cup tomato sauce

1 tsp smoked paprika

1 tsp Worcestershire sauce

⅔-cup carrots, chopped

2 1/2 cups chicken sausage, precooked and diced

4 cups lentils, soaked overnight and precooked

4 cups okra, chopped

A dash of crushed red pepper and black pepper

Directions:

1. Sauté the shrimp, celery, and fresh onion with oil in a pan placed over medium high heat for 10 minutes, or until the shrimp turn pinkish.
2. Add in the rest of the ingredients, and sauté further for 25 minutes, or until the veggies are tender.
3. To serve, divide the jambalaya mixture equally among four serving bowls. Top with pepper and cheese, if desired.

Toasted Tilapia Topped With Panko & Pecans

Ingredients:

6 tsps olive oil

4 tsps chopped fresh rosemary

A pinch of cayenne pepper

3 unit egg white

4 x 4-oz. tilapia fillets

1/7 tsp salt

1/4 cup pecans, chopped

1/4 cup whole-wheat panko breadcrumbs

1 tsp coconut palm sugar

Directions:

1. Preheat your oven to 480 °F.
2. Stir in the first seven ingredients in a small baking dish. Mix well until thoroughly combined.
3. Put the dish in the oven. Bake for 8 minutes or until the mixture turns brown. Set aside.
4. Increase the heat to 400°F. Meanwhile, grease a large baking dish with cooking spray.
5. Whisk the egg white in a shallow bowl.
6. Dip the fillet, one at a time, in the bowl of whisked egg. Dredge the soaked fillet in the pecan mixture, coating each side lightly.
7. Place each coated fillet in the large baking dish.
8. Put the dish in the oven, and bake for 25 minutes, or until the fillets cook through.

Tortilla Tostadas With Peppered Potato & Kingly Kale

Ingredients:

A pinch of salt

30 pcs Brussels sprouts, finely chopped

3 tsp honey

3 Tbsp lime juice

Corn tortillas

A drizzle of yogurt

4 pcs medium sweet potatoes, cleaned and chopped

A pinch of cayenne pepper

4 -Tbsps olive oil (divided)

8-stems kale, roughly chopped

Directions:

1. Preheat your oven to 400°F. Line two baking sheets with aluminum foil.
2. Toss the sweet potatoes with cayenne pepper and 4 tablespoons of oil on the first baking sheet.
3. In the other baking sheet, toss the kale with salt and oil.
4. Put both sheets in the oven. Roast the potatoes for 45 minutes. Roast the kale for 25 minutes until, or until the edges turn crispy, but not browned.
5. Meanwhile, toss the sprouts with the honey and lime juice. Set aside.
6. Place the corn tortillas on a piece of tin foil, and toast in the warm oven for 8 minutes.
7. To serve, scoop equally the sweet potatoes and crispy kale among four tortillas. Top each tortilla with the sprout's slaw. Drizzle with yogurt, mint, and toasted coconut, if desired.

Vanilla Turmeric Orange Juice

Ingredients:

2 teaspoon vanilla extract

1 teaspoon cinnamon

1/2 teaspoon turmeric

a pinch of pepper

4 oranges, peeled and quartered

2 cup almond milk, unsweetened

Directions:

1. Place all ingredients in a blender. Pulse until smooth.

2. Put into glasses, then chill in the fridge before serving.

Hibiscus Ginger Gelatin

Ingredients:

2 teaspoon ginger juice

2 tablespoons gelatin powder

2 cup of water

4 tablespoons dried hibiscus flower

7 tablespoon honey

Directions:
1. Boil water, remove, then add the hibiscus flowers. Allow infusing for 6 minutes.
2. Remove the flowers and discard them. Heat the liquid and add the honey, ginger, and gelatin.

3. Allow the gelatin to dissolve. Pour the mixture into a baking sheet.
4. Chill, and allow to set. Slice the gelatin once it hardens.

Buckwheat And Sweet Potatoes

Ingredients

Buckwheat groats - 1 cup

Lentils – 2 cup, rinsed

Vegetable broth – 6 cups Salt - 2 tsp.

Ground black pepper – 1 tsp.

Chopped kale – 2 cups, stemmed

Coconut oil - 2 Tbsp.

Cubed sweet potatoes – 2 cups

Yellow fresh onion – 2, chopped

Garlic – 2 cloves, minced

Ground cumin - 2 tsps.

Directions:

1. Melt the coconut oil in a pot.
2. Stir in the fresh onion ,
3. sweet potatoes, garlic, and cumin. Sauté for 6 minutes.
4. Add the lentils, buckwheat groats, vegetable broth, salt, and pepper. Bring to a boil.
5. Reduce the heat to simmer and cover the pot.
6. Cook for 35 minutes, or until the sweet potatoes, buckwheat, and lentils are tender.
7. Remove the pot from the heat.
8. Add the kale and stir to combine.
9. Cover the pot and let it sit for 10 minutes.

Zucchini Patties

Scallion – 2 , chopped

Chopped fresh mint – 2 Tbsp.

Salt – 1 tsp.

Extra-virgin olive oil - 2 Tbsps.

Medium zucchinis – 2, shredded

Salt – 2 tsp. divided

Fresh eggs – 2

Chickpea flour – 2 Tbsps.

Directions:

1. Place the shredded Zucchi in a strainer and sprinkle it with 1 tsp. salt. Set aside to drain.

2. In a bowl, beat together the chickpea flour, fresh eggs, scallion, mint, and remaining 1 tsp. salt
3. Squeeze the zucchini to remove the liquid and add it to the egg mixture. Mix well.
4. Place a large skillet over medium heat and add the olive oil.
5. Drop the zucchini mixture by spoonfuls into the pan. Gently flatten the zucchini with the back of a spatula.
6. Cook until golden brown, about 2 to 4 minutes. Flip and cook for 2 minutes more.

Shrimp Mix

2 green fresh onion , chopped

2 tablespoon balsamic vinegar

2 garlic cloves, minced

2 tablespoon ginger, grated

2 and 1 pounds shrimp, peeled and deveined

2 tablespoon essential organic olive oil

2 teaspoon sesame seeds

30 ounces broccoli florets

Directions:

1. In a bowl, mix oil with vinegar, garlic and ginger and whisk.
2. Transfer this to your pan, heat over medium heat, add shrimp, stir and cook for 8 minutes.

3. Add broccoli, stir, cook for 4 minutes more,
4. Add sesame seeds and green fresh onion s, toss, divide everything between plates and serve.

Spinach And Lentils Stew

Ingredients:

2 tomatoes, chopped

1 teaspoon turmeric powder

2 potatoes, cubed

A pinch of black pepper

1/2 teaspoon cinnamon powder

2 cup low-sodium veggie 2 teaspoon olive oil

1/2 cup brown lentils

2 teaspoon ginger, grated

4 garlic cloves, minced

2 green chili pepper, chopped

stock

6 ounces spinach leaves

Directions:

1. Heat up a pot while using oil over medium heat, add chili pepper, ginger and garlic, stir and cook for 4 minutes.
2. Add tomatoes, pepper, cinnamon, turmeric, lentils, potatoes, stock and spinach, stir and cook for 25 mins. Divide into bowls and serve. Enjoy!

Sweet Potato Mix

Ingredients:

2 teaspoons curry powder

A pinch of black pepper

2 tablespoons red curry paste

30 ounces coconut milk Juice of 4 limes

2 tablespoon cilantro, chopped

2 small yellow fresh onion , chopped

2 tablespoon essential essential olive oil

2 garlic cloves, minced

4 sweet potatoes, chopped

2 red bell pepper, chopped

30 ounces canned tomatoes, chopped

Directions:

1. Heat up a pot while using oil over medium heat, add fresh onion , stir and cook for 10 minutes.
2. Add garlic, ginger, sweet potatoes, red bell pepper, tomatoes, curry powder, and black pepper, curry paste, coconut milk, lime juice and cilantro, stir and simmer over medium heat for 25 minutes.
3. Divide into bowls and serve for lunch. Enjoy!

Pea Stew

Ingredients:

1/2 teaspoon chili powder

A pinch of black pepper

1/2 teaspoon cinnamon powder

1 cup tomatoes, chopped

Juice of 1 fresh Lemon

3 quart low-sodium veggie stock

2 tablespoon chives, chopped

2 carrot, cubed

2 yellow fresh onion , chopped

2 and 1 tablespoons essential extra virgin olive oil

2 celery stick, chopped

6 garlic cloves, minced   2 cups yellow peas

2 and 1 teaspoons cumin, ground

2 teaspoon sweet paprika

Directions:

1. Heat up a pot using the oil over medium heat, add carrots, fresh onion and celery, stir and cook for 6 - 6 minutes.
2. Add garlic, peas, cumin, paprika, chili powder, pepper, cinnamon, and tomatoes, fresh fresh Lemon juice, peas and stock, stir, bring to many simmer, cook over medium heat for twenty or so minutes, add chives, toss, divide into bowls and serve. Enjoy!

Green Beans Stew

Ingredients:

8 ounces canned tomatoes, chopped

6 cups low-sodium veggie stock

A pinch of black pepper

2 tablespoon parsley, chopped

2 tablespoons essential olive oil

2 carrots, chopped 2 yellow fresh onion , chopped

25 ounces green beans 2 garlic cloves, minced

Directions:

1. Heat up a pot while using oil, over medium heat, add fresh onion , stir and cook for 10 minutes.
2. Add carrots, green beans, garlic, tomatoes, black pepper and stock, stir, cover and simmer over medium heat for 35 approximately minutes. Add parsley, divide into bowls and serve for lunch.

Chickpeas Salad

Ingredients:

4 spring fresh onion s, chopped

2 teaspoon chili powder

2 teaspoon cumin, ground

2 tablespoon parsley, chopped

A pinch of salt and black pepper

2 cups canned chickpeas, drained and rinsed

2 tablespoon capers, chopped

2 tablespoons lime juice

2 tablespoons olive oil

Directions:

1. In a bowl, combine the chickpeas with the capers and the other ingredients, toss and serve as a side salad.

Quinoa And Beans

Ingredients:

2 cups chicken stock

2 garlic cloves, minced

Salt and black pepper to the taste

2 tablespoon cilantro, chopped

2 tablespoon olive oil

2 yellow fresh onion , chopped 2 cup quinoa

1 cup canned black beans, drained and rinsed

Directions:

2. Heat up a pan with the olive oil over medium heat, add the fresh onion and the garlic and sauté for 10 minutes.
3. Add the quinoa and the other ingredients, toss, bring to a simmer and cook over medium heat for 35 minutes.
4. Divide everything between plates and serve.

Cucumber And Green Fresh Onion S Salad

Ingredients:

1 cup cilantro, chopped

1 cup fresh Lemon juice

Salt and black pepper to the taste

2 tablespoons olive oil

2 cucumbers, sliced

4 spring fresh onion s, chopped

Directions:

1. In a salad bowl, combine the cucumbers with the spring fresh onion s and the other ingredients, toss and serve.

Barley And Kale

Ingredients:

2 tablespoons balsamic vinegar

2 tablespoon olive oil

2 tablespoon cilantro, chopped

2 cups barley, cooked

2 cup baby kale

2 tablespoons almonds, chopped

Directions:

1. In a bowl, mix the barley with the kale, the almonds and the other ingredients, toss and serve as a side dish.

Herbed Mango Mix

Ingredients:

2 tablespoon olive oil

2 tablespoon chives, chopped

2 tablespoon oregano, chopped

2 tablespoon basil, chopped

2 tablespoons fresh Lemon juice

Salt and black pepper to the taste

2 mangos, peeled and chopped

2 spring fresh onion s, chopped

2 avocado, peeled, pitted and cubed

Directions:

1. In a salad bowl, mix the mangos with the spring fresh onion s, the avocado and the other ingredients, toss and serve as a side dish.

Cabbage Slaw

Ingredients:

2 tablespoon fresh Lemon juice

2 garlic cloves, minced

2 tablespoon apple cider vinegar

4 tablespoons olive oil

2 tablespoon parsley, chopped

A pinch of salt and black pepper

2 cups green cabbage, shredded

2 carrot, grated

4 dates, chopped

2 tablespoons walnuts, chopped

Directions:

1. In a bowl, combine the cabbage with the carrots, dates and the other ingredients, toss and serve as a side salad.

Cucumber With Apples Alad

Ingredients:

4 teaspoons orange juice

A pinch of salt and black pepper

2 tablespoon mint, chopped

2 tablespoon fresh Lemon juice

2 cucumbers, sliced

2 green apple, cored and cubed

4 spring fresh onion s, chopped

4 tablespoons olive oil

Directions:

1. In a bowl, mix the cucumbers with the apple, spring fresh onion s and the other ingredients, toss and serve as a side salad.

Parsley Avocado Mix

Ingredients:

2 tablespoon fresh Lemon juice

2 tablespoon fresh Lemon zest, grated

A pinch of salt and black pepper

2 tablespoon olive oil

2 avocados, peeled, pitted and sliced

2 tablespoon parsley, chopped

Directions:

1. In a bowl, combine the avocados with the oil, the parsley and the other ingredients, toss and serve as a side dish.

Endives And Broccoli

Ingredients:

2 teaspoon rosemary, dried

2 teaspoon cumin, ground

2 teaspoon chili powder

2 endives, shredded

2 cup broccoli florets

2 tablespoons olive oil

2 tablespoon walnuts, chopped

2 tablespoon almonds, chopped

2 garlic cloves, minced

Directions:

1. In a roasting pan, combine the endives with the broccoli and the other ingredients, toss and bake at 4 80 degrees F for 25 minutes.
2. Divide the mix between plates and serve.

Arugula Salad

Ingredients:

2 cups baby arugula

Juice of 2 lime

1 cup cherry tomatoes, halved

2 tablespoon olive oil

2 tablespoon balsamic vinegar

A pinch of salt and black pepper

2 tablespoon chives, chopped

Directions:

1. In a salad bowl, mix the arugula with the lime juice, cherry tomatoes and the other ingredients, toss and serve.

Morning Bowl

Ingredients:

2 teaspoon pine nuts; raw

2 teaspoon pepitas; raw

2 teaspoons raspberries

2 teaspoon pecans; chopped.

2 teaspoon sunflower seeds; raw

2 cup coconut milk

2 teaspoon raw honey

2 teaspoon walnuts; chopped.

2 teaspoon pistachios; chopped.

2 teaspoon almonds; chopped.

Directions:

1. In a bowl, mix milk with honey and stir.
2. Add pecans, walnuts, almonds, pistachios, sunflower seeds, pine nuts and pepitas
3. Stir, top with raspberries and serve

2. Breakfast Stir Fry

Ingredients:

2 teaspoon chili powder

2 tablespoon coconut oil

Salt and black pepper to the taste.

1 pounds beef meat; minced

2 tablespoon tamari sauce

2 bell peppers; chopped.

2 teaspoons red chili flakes

For the bok choy:

Salt to the taste.

For the eggs:

2 fresh eggs

2 tablespoon coconut oil

6 bunches bok choy; trimmed and chopped.

2 teaspoon ginger; grated

3 tablespoon coconut oil

Directions:

1. Heat up a pan with 2 tablespoon coconut oil over medium high heat; add beef and bell peppers; stir and cook for 25 minutes
2. Add salt, pepper, tamari sauce, chili flakes and chili powder; stir, cook for 4 minutes more and take off heat.
3. Heat up another pan with 2 tablespoon oil over medium heat; add bok choy; stir and cook for 8 minutes

4. Add salt and ginger; stir, cook for 2 minutes more and take off heat.
5. Heat up the third pan with 2 tablespoon oil over medium heat; crack fresh eggs and fry them.
6. Divide beef and bell peppers mix into 2 bowls
7. Divide bok choy and top with fresh eggs

Cereal Nibs

Ingredients:

2 tablespoons cocoa nibs

2 tablespoon vanilla extract

2 tablespoon psyllium powder

2 cup water

4 tablespoons hemp hearts

1 cup chia seeds

2 tablespoons coconut oil

2 tablespoon swerve

Directions:

1. In a bowl, mix chia seeds with water; stir and leave aside for 10 minutes
2. Add hemp hearts, vanilla extract, psyllium powder, oil and swerve and stir well with your mixer.
3. Add cocoa nibs, and stir until you obtain a dough.
4. Divide dough into 2 pieces, shape into cylinder form, place on a lined baking sheet, flatten well, cover with a parchment paper, introduce in the oven at 280 degrees F and bake for 25 minutes
5. Remove the parchment paper and bake for 35 minutes more
6. Take cylinders out of the oven, leave aside to cool down and cut into small pieces
7. Serve in the morning with some almond milk.

Chicken Muffins

Ingredients:

4 tablespoons hot sauce mixed with 4 tablespoons melted coconut oil

6 fresh eggs

Salt and black pepper to the taste.

1/2 pound chicken breast; boneless

1 teaspoon garlic powder

2 tablespoons green fresh onion s; chopped.

Directions:

1. Season chicken breast with salt, pepper and garlic powder, place on a lined baking sheet and bake in the oven at 435 degrees F for 35 minutes
2. Transfer chicken breast to a bowl, shred with a fork and mix with half of the hot sauce and melted coconut oil.
3. Toss to coat and leave aside for now.
4. In a bowl, mix fresh eggs with salt, pepper, green fresh onion s and the rest of the hot sauce mixed with oil and whisk very well.
5. Divide this mix into a muffin tray, top each with shredded chicken, introduce in the oven at 4 70 degrees F and bake for 45 minutes
6. Serve your muffins hot.

Egg Porridge

Ingredients:

2 fresh eggs

2 tablespoons ghee; melted

1/2 cup heavy cream

2 tablespoon stevia

A pinch of cinnamon; ground

Directions:

1. In a bowl, mix fresh eggs with stevia and heavy cream and whisk well.
2. Heat up a pan with the ghee over medium high heat; add egg mix and cook until they are done
3. Transfer to 2 bowls, sprinkle cinnamon on top and serve

Celery Root Hash Browns

Ingredients:

1 tsp sea salt

2 to 4 medium celery roots

4 tbsp coconut oil

Directions:

1. Scrub the celery root clean and peel it using a vegetable peeler.
2. Grate the celery root in a food processor or a manual grater.
3. In a skillet, add oil and heat it over medium heat.
4. Place the grated celery root on the skillet and sprinkle with salt.

5. Let it cook for 25 minutes on each side or until the grated celery turns brown.
6. Serve warm.

Zucchini Pasta With Avocado Sauce

Ingredients:

1 ripe avocado 2 tbsp olive oil

2 medium zucchini cut into noodles

A squeeze of fresh Lemon juice

Salt and pepper to taste 2 tbsp coconut milk

Directions:

1. Heat the oil in a skillet over medium heat and add the zucchini noodles.

Sauté for three minutes or until the noodles have softened.
2. While the zucchini is cooking, mash the avocado together with the coconut milk, fresh Lemon juice and salt and pepper. Add the sauce to the zucchini noodles and sauté. Serve warm.

Blueberry Chia Pudding

Ingredients:

1/2 cup almond milk

2 cups frozen blueberries

1 cup chia seeds

1 of frozen banana

6 dates (soaked in water)

Directions:

1. Combine the milk, blueberries, dates and bananas in a blender. Process until the mixture becomes smooth.
2. Transfer the blueberry to a bowl and add the chia seeds.

3. Refrigerate for 45 minutes or overnight if necessary, until the chia seeds forms mucilage.
4. Serve with your favorite fruit or nut toppings.

Collard Green Wrap

Ingredients:

2 cup low-fat plain Greek yogurt

2 tablespoon white vinegar

2 teaspoon garlic powder

2 tablespoons minced fresh dill

2 tablespoons olive oil

2.6 -ounces cucumber, seeded and grated (1/2 whole)

Salt and pepper to taste

1 block feta, cut into 4 (3 inch thick) strips (4-oz)

1 cup purple fresh onion , diced

1 medium red bell pepper, julienned

2 medium cucumber, julienned

4 large cherry tomatoes, halved

4 large collard green leaves, washed

8 whole kalamata olives, halved

Sauce Ingredients:

Directions:

1. Make the sauce first: make sure to squeeze out all the excess liquid from the cucumber after grating.
2. In a small bowl, mix all sauce ingredients thoroughly and refrigerate.

3. Prepare and slice all wrap ingredients.
4. On a flat surface, spread one collard green leaf. Spread 2 tablespoons of Tzatziki sauce on middle of the leaf.
5. Layer 1/2 of each of the tomatoes, feta, olives, fresh onion , pepper, and cucumber. Place them on the center of the leaf, like piling them high instead of spreading them.
6. Fold the leaf like you would a burrito. Repeat process for remaining ingredients.
7. Serve and enjoy.

Zucchini Garlic Fries

Ingredients:

2 large egg whites, beaten

4 medium zucchinis, sliced into fry sticks

Salt and pepper to taste

1/2 teaspoon garlic powder

1 cup almond flour

Directions:

1. Preheat oven to 400oF.
2. Mix all ingredients in a bowl until the zucchini fries are well coated.
3. Place fries on cookie sheet and spread evenly.
4. Put in oven and cook for 25 minutes.
5. Halfway through cooking time, stir

Mashed Cauliflower

Ingredients:

1/2 tsp dill

Pepper to taste

2 tbsp low fat milk

2 cauliflower head

2 tablespoon olive oil

1 tsp salt

Directions:

1. Bring a small pot of water to a boil.
2. Chop cauliflower in florets.
3. Add florets to boiling water and boil uncovered for 6 minutes. Turn off fire and let it sit for 10 minutes more.

4. In a blender, add all ingredients except for cauliflower and blend to mix well.
5. Drain cauliflower well and add into blender. Puree until smooth and creamy.
6. Serve and enjoy.

Conclusion

It's clear that inflammation has both advantages and disadvantages to the body system. Its positive side involves healing joints, muscles, and body pains while its terrible side results from its good sides, which includes; causing heart attacks, stroke, soreness, and swelling, among others. Since a lot of prevention and treatment techniques have been discussed in the cookbook, everyone needs to understand their inflammation status.

Also, the anti-inflammation recipes compiled in this book are delicious, healthy, and easy to prepare. We have also simplified your shopping hassle by preparing a pantry list. You can begin by following our recipes and meal plans. After getting used, plan your dieting and modify your favorite dishes using anti-inflammatory ingredients. Note the number of servings before preparing any recipe for a balanced diet.

Inflammation of a body part is, in fact, the response given by the immune system to unfavorable stimuli like infections, damaged cells, and tissues, various pathogens, etThough this process is natural and quite harmless, it is something to worry about if the inflammation is persistent and chroniIn such cases it can do more harm than good and worsen the affected area.

The digestive tract or the gut is one of the most common sites of inflammation as a lot of pathogens enter the digestive system through the food we eat. Though the problem is not severe in most individuals, there are a lot of people who suffer from chronic inflammation. These recipes here will not only help to nullify the inflammation to a great extent but will also prevent further damage as well.

Inflammation has to be regarded as a serious condition, which can lead to devastating effects on your health. By reading this book, you have gained more knowledge about acute or chronic inflammation, and also about their causes. Although in some cases more research is required, most of us can agree that inflammatory conditions can be prevented and even reversed. Probably you are not very convinced about the power of diets when it comes to health benefits, but by acknowledging the danger of inflammation and the benefits of anti-inflammatory foods, you should consider the meal plan presented in this book.

However, everyone should be cautious about their body health before taking vitamins, supplements, and the creams discussed to avoid more repercussions. Remember to seek your doctor's help before consuming them, and immediately you note any side effect after taking them.

www.ingramcontent.com/pod-product-compliance
Lightning Source LLC
LaVergne TN
LVHW011950070526
838202LV00054B/4885